DIABETIC RENAL DIET COOKBOOK

DELICIOUS AND HEALTHY RECIPES FOR MANAGING DIABETES AND KIDNEY DISEASE

VICTOR S. OSBORNE, MD

DISCLAIMER

The recipes and information in this cookbook are intended for general informational and educational purposes only. They are not intended to be a substitute for professional medical advice, diagnosis, or treatment. Always seek the advice of your healthcare professional or registered dietitian before making any changes to your diet or exercise routine. The authors and publisher of this cookbook are not responsible for any adverse effects or consequences resulting from the use of the information contained in this cookbook.

TABLE OF CONTENT

TABLE OF CONTENT 4

DEDICATION 8

PREFACE 10

CHAPTER I: 12

INTRODUCTION TO THE DIABETIC RENAL DIET 12

Why is the Diabetic Renal Diet Important? 14

What Does the Diabetic Renal Diet Involve? 15

Tips for Following a Diabetic Renal Diet 18

CHAPTER II: 22

MEAL PLANNING AND PORTION CONTROL 22

Importance of Meal Planning for Blood Sugar Management 24

How to Portion Out Meals and Snacks 26

Tips for Eating Out and Making Healthy Choices 27

CHAPTER III: **30**

RECIPES   **30**

OMELETTE WITH VEGETABLES AND LOW-FAT CHEESE   32

SAUSAGE AND EGG MUFFINS WITH WHOLE-GRAIN ENGLISH MUFFINS 36

SMOOTHIE WITH BANANA, BERRIES, AND ALMOND MILK   40

WHOLE GRAIN CEREAL WITH MILK AND FRUIT   43

GRILLED CHICKEN AND VEGETABLE SKEWERS WITH QUINOA   46

BAKED TURKEY AND VEGETABLE MEATBALLS WITH WHOLE GRAIN SPAGHETTI   50

ROASTED SALMON WITH SWEET POTATO AND BROCCOLI   55

GRILLED SHRIMP WITH CORN AND BLACK BEAN SALAD   59

VEGETABLE AND BEAN SOUP WITH WHOLE GRAIN BREAD   63

BAKED CHICKEN WITH QUINOA AND ROASTED VEGETABLES   67

GRILLED TURKEY AND VEGETABLE WRAP WITH WHOLE GRAIN TORTILLA 71

WHOLE GRAIN PASTA WITH TOMATO SAUCE AND STEAMED VEGETABLES 76

SLOW COOKER VEGETABLE AND BEAN CHILI WITH WHOLE GRAIN CORNBREAD 80

GRILLED PORK CHOP WITH ROASTED POTATOES AND ASPARAGUS 86

BAKED TOFU WITH BROWN RICE AND STIR-FRIED VEGETABLES 90

GRILLED CHICKEN CAESAR SALAD WITH WHOLE GRAIN CROUTONS 95

TURKEY AND VEGETABLE STIR-FRY WITH BROWN RICE 99

SLOW COOKER BEEF AND VEGETABLE STEW WITH WHOLE GRAIN BISCUITS 103

GRILLED SALMON WITH QUINOA AND ROASTED VEGETABLES 108

BAKED CHICKEN WITH MASHED SWEET POTATOES AND GREEN BEANS 113

WHOLE GRAIN PIZZA WITH VEGETABLES AND LOW-FAT CHEESE 118

GRILLED CHICKEN AND AVOCADO SALAD WITH MIXED GREENS 122

SLOW COOKER CHICKEN AND VEGETABLE SOUP WITH WHOLE GRAIN BREAD 127

BAKED TILAPIA WITH QUINOA AND STEAMED BROCCOLI 132

GRILLED PORK WITH ROASTED SWEET POTATO AND BRUSSELS SPROUTS 137

VEGETABLE AND BEAN BURRITOS WITH WHOLE GRAIN TORTILLAS 141

GRILLED CHICKEN AND VEGETABLE SKEWERS WITH BROWN RICE 145

BAKED TURKEY MEATLOAF WITH MASHED SWEET POTATOES AND GREEN BEANS 150

GRILLED SALMON WITH QUINOA AND ROASTED ASPARAGUS 155

CONCLUSION **160**

DEDICATION

To all the warriors out there fighting diabetes and kidney disease every day: this book is dedicated to you. Your strength, courage, and determination inspire us all.

Living with chronic conditions is not easy, but you face each day with grace and resilience. You are a source of hope and inspiration to those around you, and we are honored to be a part of your journey.

May this cookbook be a source of comfort, inspiration, and delicious meals as you navigate the ups and downs of managing your health. You are not alone, and you are loved.

PREFACE

Welcome to our Diabetic Renal Diet Cookbook! If you're reading this, chances are you or someone you love is living with diabetes and kidney disease. Managing both of these conditions can be a challenge, but it's important to remember that you are not alone.

There are millions of people all over the world who are successfully managing their diabetes and kidney disease, and with the right tools and resources, you can too.

That's where this cookbook comes in. Inside these pages, you'll find a collection of delicious and healthy recipes that have been carefully crafted to help you manage your diabetes and kidney disease. From breakfast dishes to main courses to desserts, we've got you covered. But this book is about more than just recipes. It's about empowering you to take control of your health and live a full and rewarding life.

So, let's get cooking!

Whether you're a seasoned chef or a beginner, we hope these recipes will inspire you to get creative in the kitchen and make mealtime enjoyable again. Remember, your health is worth the effort, and every small step you take towards better management of your diabetes and kidney disease can make a big difference.

Happy cooking!

CHAPTER I:

INTRODUCTION TO THE DIABETIC RENAL DIET

The diabetic renal diet is a special type of meal plan that is designed for individuals with both diabetes and kidney disease. This diet helps to manage blood sugar levels, reduce the risk of complications, and protect the kidneys from further damage.

Why is the Diabetic Renal Diet Important?

Diabetes is a chronic condition that affects the way the body processes sugar (glucose). It occurs when the body either does not produce enough insulin (a hormone that helps regulate blood sugar levels) or does not use insulin properly. This can lead to high levels of sugar in the blood, which can damage the blood vessels and organs over time.

Kidney disease is a condition that occurs when the kidneys are damaged and cannot filter waste products and excess fluids from the blood effectively. This can lead to a buildup of toxins in the body and can cause a number of complications, including high blood pressure, anemia, and nerve damage.

Individuals with both diabetes and kidney disease have an increased risk of developing complications, such as heart disease, nerve damage, and anemia. The diabetic renal diet is designed to help manage blood sugar levels and protect the kidneys from further damage.

What Does the Diabetic Renal Diet Involve?

The diabetic renal diet typically involves:

- Limiting salt intake: High levels of salt can put additional strain on the kidneys and increase the risk of high blood pressure. It is recommended to aim for less than 2,000 milligrams (mg) of sodium per day.

- Limiting protein intake: High levels of protein can put additional strain on the kidneys. It is important to get enough protein to maintain muscle mass, but not too much that it puts excess strain on the kidneys. A registered dietitian can help determine the appropriate amount of protein for an individual's specific needs.

- Limiting saturated and trans fats: These types of fats can increase the risk of heart disease, which is a common complication in individuals with diabetes and kidney disease. It is recommended to choose sources of fat that are high in monounsaturated and polyunsaturated fats, such as olive oil, nuts, and avocados.

- Choosing complex carbohydrates: Complex carbohydrates, such as whole grains, fruits, and vegetables, are less likely to cause spikes in blood sugar levels. It is recommended to choose these types of carbohydrates over refined, sugary sources.

- Monitoring portion sizes: Proper portion control is important for managing blood sugar levels and maintaining a healthy weight. A registered dietitian can help determine the appropriate portion sizes for an individual's specific needs.

- Reading food labels: It is important to be aware of the nutritional content of the foods that are being consumed. Reading food labels can help individuals make informed choices about what to eat.

Tips for Following a Diabetic Renal Diet

1. Work with a registered dietitian: A registered dietitian can help develop an individualized meal plan that meets an individual's specific needs and health goals.

2. Plan ahead: Meal planning and preparing food in advance can make it easier to stick to the diabetic renal diet.

3. Keep a food diary: Keeping track of what is being eaten can help identify any potential issues or areas for improvement in the diet.

4. Be mindful of portion sizes: It is important to pay attention to portion sizes to help manage blood sugar levels and maintain a healthy weight.

5. Choose healthy fats: Choose sources of fat that are high in monounsaturated and polyunsaturated fats, such as olive oil, nuts, and avocados.

6. Get support: It can be helpful to enlist the support of family and friends to help stay on track with the diabetic renal diet. Joining a support group or working with a nutritionist or dietitian can also be helpful.

7. Make healthy swaps: It is possible to still enjoy your favorite foods while following the diabetic renal diet. Try making healthy swaps, such as using whole-grain bread instead of white bread or substituting Greek yogurt for sour cream.

By following the diabetic renal diet and working with a healthcare team, individuals with diabetes and kidney disease can better manage their condition and reduce the risk of complications.

CHAPTER II:

MEAL PLANNING AND PORTION CONTROL

P

roper meal planning and portion control are important components of the diabetic renal diet. This chapter will cover the importance of meal planning for blood sugar management, how to portion out meals and snacks, and tips for eating out and making healthy choices.

Importance of Meal Planning for Blood Sugar Management

Meal planning involves organizing and preparing meals and snacks in advance to ensure that they meet the nutritional needs of the individual. This can be especially important for individuals with diabetes, as it helps to manage blood sugar levels and reduce the risk of complications.

Some benefits of meal planning for individuals with diabetes include:

1. Better blood sugar control: Meal planning allows individuals to control the types and amounts of foods that are consumed, which can help manage blood sugar levels.

2. Weight management: Meal planning can help individuals maintain a healthy weight, which can improve blood sugar control and reduce the risk of complications.

3. Reducing stress: Planning meals in advance can save time and reduce stress, as individuals do not need to worry about what to eat on a daily basis.

4. Improving nutrition: Meal planning allows individuals to ensure that they are meeting their nutritional needs and getting the right balance of nutrients.

How to Portion Out Meals and Snacks

Proper portion control is important for managing blood sugar levels and maintaining a healthy weight. A registered dietitian can help determine the appropriate portion sizes for an individual's specific needs.

Here are some general guidelines for portion sizes:

- Grains: 1 serving = 1 slice of bread, 1 cup of cereal, or 1/2 cup of cooked grains (such as rice or pasta)

- Vegetables: 1 serving = 1 cup of raw vegetables, 1/2 cup of cooked vegetables, or 1/2 cup of vegetable juice

- Fruits: 1 serving = 1 medium fruit, 1/2 cup of chopped fruit, or 1/2 cup of fruit juice

- Proteins: 1 serving = 3 ounces of cooked meat, poultry, or fish; 1/2 cup of cooked beans; or 2 tablespoons of nut butter

- Fats: 1 serving = 1 teaspoon of oil, 1 tablespoon of nut butter, or 1/3 cup of nuts

Tips for Eating Out and Making Healthy Choices

Eating out can be challenging for individuals following a diabetic renal diet, as it is often difficult to know the nutritional content of the foods being served. Here are some tips for making healthy choices when eating out:

1. Choose restaurants that offer healthy options: Look for restaurants that have a variety of healthy options, such as salads, grilled meats, and steamed vegetables.

2. Ask about preparation methods: Ask how the food is prepared and request that it be cooked without added salt or fat.

3. Share dishes: Consider sharing a dish with a friend or taking half of the meal home for leftovers.

4. Make smart substitutions: Substitute a side salad or vegetables for French fries, and choose water or unsweetened tea instead of soda.

By incorporating proper meal planning and portion control into the diabetic renal diet, individuals can better manage their blood sugar levels and reduce the risk of complications. It is important to work with a registered dietitian to determine the appropriate meal plan and portion sizes for an individual's specific needs.

CHAPTER III:

RECIPES

OMELETTE WITH VEGETABLES AND LOW-FAT CHEESE

Servings: 1

Ingredients:

- 2 large eggs
- 1/4 cup diced bell peppers
- 1/4 cup diced onions
- 1/4 cup diced tomatoes
- 1/4 cup diced zucchini
- 1/4 cup low-fat shredded cheese (such as mozzarella or cheddar)
- 1 teaspoon olive oil
- Salt and pepper, to taste

Instructions:

1. Crack the eggs into a bowl and whisk lightly. Set aside.
2. Heat a non-stick skillet over medium heat. Add the olive oil and let it warm up.

3. Add the diced bell peppers, onions, tomatoes, and zucchini to the skillet. Sauté for 2-3 minutes, or until the vegetables are slightly tender.

4. Pour the eggs over the vegetables in the skillet. Season with salt and pepper, to taste.

5. Let the eggs cook for 1-2 minutes, or until the edges start to set. Using a spatula, gently lift the edges of the omelette and tilt the skillet to allow the uncooked egg to flow underneath.

6. When the eggs are almost fully cooked, sprinkle the low-fat cheese over one half of the omelette.

7. Carefully fold the omelette in half, using the spatula to help lift and fold it.

8. Let the omelette cook for an additional 30 seconds to 1 minute, or until the cheese is melted and the omelette is fully cooked.

9. Remove the omelette from the skillet and serve immediately.

Health Benefits:

This omelette is a great source of protein and vitamins thanks to the eggs and vegetables. The protein in eggs can help keep you feeling full and satisfied, while the vegetables provide a variety of essential vitamins and minerals.
The use of low-fat cheese in this recipe helps to reduce the overall fat and calorie content, making it a healthier choice than a traditional omelette made with full-fat cheese.

Nutritional Information (per serving):

- Calories: 200
- Total Fat: 12 g
- Saturated Fat: 4 g
- Cholesterol: 372 mg
- Sodium: 358 mg
- Total Carbohydrates: 8 g
- Dietary Fiber: 2 g

- Protein: 16 g

Substitutions:

1. If you don't have bell peppers, onions, tomatoes, or zucchini on hand, feel free to use any other vegetables you have on hand. Some options could include diced mushrooms, spinach, or asparagus.
2. If you're not a fan of low-fat cheese, you can use any type of cheese that you prefer. Just keep in mind that using full-fat cheese will increase the calorie and fat content of the omelette.
3. If you're trying to avoid eggs, you can try using a plant-based egg substitute in this recipe. Just follow the instructions on the package to prepare the egg substitute and use it in place of the eggs in this recipe.

SAUSAGE AND EGG MUFFINS WITH WHOLE-GRAIN ENGLISH MUFFINS

Servings: 4

Ingredients:

- 4 whole-grain English muffins
- 8 turkey sausage patties
- 8 large eggs
- Salt and pepper, to taste

Instructions:

1. Preheat your oven to 350°F (180°C).
2. Cut the turkey sausage patties into small pieces and set aside.
3. Crack the eggs into a bowl and whisk lightly. Season with salt and pepper, to taste.
4. Toast the English muffins until they are slightly crispy.

5. Once toasted, place the English muffins on a baking sheet.
6. Top each English muffin with a few pieces of sausage and then pour the eggs over the sausage on each muffin.
7. Bake the muffins in the preheated oven for 10-12 minutes, or until the eggs are cooked through.
8. Serve the muffins immediately.

Health Benefits:

These muffins are a convenient and portable breakfast option that is high in protein thanks to the eggs and turkey sausage. Protein is important for maintaining muscle mass and can help keep you feeling full and satisfied.

The use of whole-grain English muffins in this recipe adds some fiber to the dish, which can help support healthy digestion.

Nutritional Information (per serving):

- Calories: 280
- Total Fat: 14 g
- Saturated Fat: 4 g
- Cholesterol: 220 mg
- Sodium: 830 mg
- Total Carbohydrates: 22 g
- Dietary Fiber: 3 g
- Protein: 17 g

Substitutions:

1. If you don't have turkey sausage on hand, you can use any type of sausage that you prefer. Just keep in mind that using a sausage with a higher fat content will increase the calorie and fat content of the muffins.
2. If you're trying to reduce the fat content of this recipe, you can use egg whites instead of whole eggs. Just be sure to adjust the cooking time as

needed since egg whites cook faster than whole eggs.

3. If you're not a fan of English muffins, you can use any type of bread or muffin that you prefer. Just keep in mind that using a different type of bread or muffin may affect the nutritional information.

SMOOTHIE WITH BANANA, BERRIES, AND ALMOND MILK

Servings: 1

Ingredients:

- 1 banana
- 1 cup frozen berries (such as strawberries, blueberries, or raspberries)
- 1 cup unsweetened almond milk
- 1 teaspoon honey (optional)

Instructions:

1. Peel the banana and cut it into small pieces.
2. Place the banana, frozen berries, almond milk, and honey (if using) in a blender.
3. Blend the ingredients on high speed until the smoothie is smooth and creamy, about 30-60 seconds.

4. Pour the smoothie into a glass and serve immediately.

Health Benefits:

This smoothie is a great source of vitamins and minerals thanks to the banana and berries. Bananas are a good source of potassium, which is important for maintaining healthy blood pressure, and berries are high in antioxidants, which can help protect against cell damage.
Almond milk is a good source of calcium, which is important for maintaining strong bones, and is also lower in calories and fat compared to cow's milk.

Nutritional Information (per serving):

- Calories: 160
- Total Fat: 2.5 g
- Saturated Fat: 0 g
- Cholesterol: 0 mg

- Sodium: 180 mg
- Total Carbohydrates: 34 g
- Dietary Fiber: 4 g
- Protein: 2 g

Substitutions:

1. If you don't have frozen berries on hand, you can use fresh berries and add a few ice cubes to the blender to help thicken the smoothie.
2. If you're not a fan of almond milk, you can use any type of milk that you prefer. Just keep in mind that using a different type of milk may affect the nutritional information.
3. If you don't have honey, you can use any type of sweetener that you prefer, such as maple syrup or agave nectar. You can also omit the sweetener altogether if you prefer a less sweet smoothie.

WHOLE GRAIN CEREAL WITH MILK AND FRUIT

Servings: 1

Ingredients:

- 1 cup whole grain cereal (such as oats, quinoa flakes, or whole grain flakes)
- 1 cup unsweetened almond milk (or any type of milk you prefer)
- 1/2 cup fresh fruit (such as berries, sliced bananas, or diced apples)

Instructions:

1. Pour the cereal into a bowl.
2. Add the almond milk to the bowl and stir until the cereal is fully coated.
3. Top the cereal with the fresh fruit.
4. Serve the cereal immediately.

Health Benefits:

This cereal is a good source of whole grains, which are important for maintaining good digestive health and can help support a healthy heart.
The almond milk provides a good source of calcium, which is important for maintaining strong bones, and is also lower in calories and fat compared to cow's milk.
The fresh fruit adds a boost of vitamins and minerals to the dish, as well as some natural sweetness.

Nutritional Information (per serving):

- Calories: 250
- Total Fat: 5 g
- Saturated Fat: 0.5 g
- Cholesterol: 0 mg
- Sodium: 180 mg
- Total Carbohydrates: 46 g
- Dietary Fiber: 6 g

- Protein: 8 g

Substitutions:

1. If you don't have any whole-grain cereal on hand, you can use any type of cereal that you prefer. Just keep in mind that using a cereal that is not made with whole grains will not provide the same health benefits.
2. If you're not a fan of almond milk, you can use any type of milk that you prefer. Just keep in mind that using a different type of milk may affect the nutritional information.
3. If you don't have any fresh fruit on hand, you can use frozen fruit or dried fruit instead. You can also omit the fruit altogether if you prefer.

GRILLED CHICKEN AND VEGETABLE SKEWERS WITH QUINOA

Servings: 4

Ingredients:

- 1 pound boneless, skinless chicken breasts, cut into 1-inch pieces
- 2 bell peppers, cut into 1-inch pieces
- 2 medium zucchini, cut into 1-inch pieces
- 1 medium onion, cut into 1-inch pieces
- 1 cup cherry tomatoes
- 2 tablespoons olive oil
- Salt and pepper, to taste
- 1 cup uncooked quinoa
- 2 cups water

Instructions:

1. Preheat your grill to medium-high heat.
2. Thread the chicken, bell peppers, zucchini, onion, and cherry tomatoes onto skewers.
3. Brush the skewers with olive oil and season with salt and pepper, to taste.
4. Place the skewers on the grill and cook for 8-10 minutes, or until the chicken is cooked through and the vegetables are tender, turning occasionally.
5. Meanwhile, rinse the quinoa in a fine mesh strainer.
6. In a medium saucepan, bring the water to a boil. Add the quinoa and reduce the heat to low.
7. Cover the saucepan and simmer for 15-20 minutes, or until the quinoa is tender and the water is absorbed.
8. Fluff the quinoa with a fork and serve it alongside the grilled chicken and vegetable skewers.

Health Benefits:

This dish is a good source of protein thanks to the chicken and quinoa. Protein is important for maintaining muscle mass and can help keep you feeling full and satisfied.

The vegetables provide a variety of essential vitamins and minerals, as well as fiber, which is important for maintaining good digestive health.

Quinoa is a good source of whole grains, which are important for maintaining good digestive health and can help support a healthy heart.

Nutritional Information (per serving):

- Calories: 310
- Total Fat: 8 g
- Saturated Fat: 1 g
- Cholesterol: 45 mg

- Sodium: 120 mg
- Total Carbohydrates: 41 g
- Dietary Fiber: 5 g
- Protein: 20 g

Substitutions:

1. If you don't have chicken on hand, you can use any type of protein that you prefer, such as tofu, shrimp, or beef. Just keep in mind that using a different type of protein may affect the nutritional information.
2. If you don't have bell peppers, zucchini, or onion on hand, you can use any type of vegetable that you prefer. Some options could include mushrooms, asparagus, or eggplant.
3. If you're not a fan of quinoa, you can use any type of grain that you prefer, such as brown rice, wild rice, or farro. Just keep in mind that using a different type of grain may affect the nutritional information.

BAKED TURKEY AND VEGETABLE MEATBALLS WITH WHOLE GRAIN SPAGHETTI

Servings: 4

Ingredients:

- 1 pound ground turkey
- 1 cup grated zucchini
- 1/2 cup grated carrot
- 1/4 cup grated parmesan cheese
- 1/4 cup whole wheat breadcrumbs
- 1 egg
- 1 clove garlic, minced
- 1 teaspoon Italian seasoning
- Salt and pepper, to taste
- 1 tablespoon olive oil
- 1 pound whole grain spaghetti
- 1 jar marinara sauce

Instructions:

1. Preheat your oven to 400°F (200°C).
2. In a large bowl, combine the ground turkey, grated zucchini, grated carrot, parmesan cheese, breadcrumbs, egg, minced garlic, Italian seasoning, salt, and pepper. Mix until well combined.
3. Shape the mixture into small meatballs (about the size of a golf ball) and place them on a baking sheet lined with parchment paper.
4. Brush the meatballs with olive oil and bake them in the preheated oven for 20-25 minutes, or until they are cooked through and browned on the outside.
5. Meanwhile, bring a large pot of salted water to a boil. Add the spaghetti and cook it according to the package instructions until it is al dente.
6. Drain the spaghetti and return it to the pot. Add the marinara sauce and stir to combine.

7. Serve the spaghetti and meatballs hot, with additional grated parmesan cheese on top if desired.

Health Benefits:

This dish is a good source of protein thanks to the turkey and whole grain spaghetti. Protein is important for maintaining muscle mass and can help keep you feeling full and satisfied. The whole grain spaghetti provides some additional fiber, which is important for maintaining good digestive health.

The vegetables in the meatballs (zucchini and carrot) provide a variety of essential vitamins and minerals, as well as adding some moisture to the meatballs.

Nutritional Information (per serving):

- Calories: 450

- Total Fat: 11 g
- Saturated Fat: 3 g
- Cholesterol: 95 mg
- Sodium: 550 mg
- Total Carbohydrates: 60 g
- Dietary Fiber: 6 g
- Protein: 30 g

Substitutions:

1. If you don't have ground turkey on hand, you can use any type of ground meat that you prefer, such as beef, chicken, or pork. Just keep in mind that using a different type of meat may affect the nutritional information.
2. If you don't have whole grain spaghetti on hand, you can use any type of pasta that you prefer. Just keep in mind that using a pasta that is not made with whole grains will not provide the same health benefits.

3. If you don't have zucchini or carrot on hand, you can use any type of grated vegetables that you prefer, such as bell peppers, mushrooms, or eggplant. You can also omit the vegetables altogether if you prefer.

4. If you don't have marinara sauce on hand, you can use any type of tomato-based sauce that you prefer, such as a vodka sauce or a arrabbiata sauce. You can also make your own sauce by simmering diced tomatoes with some garlic, olive oil, and herbs.

ROASTED SALMON WITH SWEET POTATO AND BROCCOLI

Servings: 4

Ingredients:

- 4 (4-ounce) salmon fillets
- 2 medium sweet potatoes, cut into 1-inch pieces
- 1 large head broccoli, cut into florets
- 2 tablespoons olive oil
- Salt and pepper, to taste

Instructions:

1. Preheat your oven to 400°F (200°C).
2. Place the sweet potatoes on one side of a large baking sheet and the broccoli on the other side.
3. Brush the sweet potatoes and broccoli with olive oil and season with salt and pepper, to taste.

4. Place the salmon fillets on top of the broccoli.
5. Roast the vegetables and salmon in the preheated oven for 15-20 minutes, or until the salmon is cooked through and the vegetables are tender.
6. Serve the salmon with the sweet potato and broccoli on the side.

Health Benefits:

This dish is a good source of protein thanks to the salmon. Protein is important for maintaining muscle mass and can help keep you feeling full and satisfied.

The sweet potatoes and broccoli provide a variety of essential vitamins and minerals, as well as fiber, which is important for maintaining good digestive health.

Salmon is a good source of omega-3 fatty acids, which are important for maintaining heart health.

Nutritional Information (per serving):

- Calories: 250
- Total Fat: 9 g
- Saturated Fat: 1.5 g
- Cholesterol: 70 mg
- Sodium: 90 mg
- Total Carbohydrates: 23 g
- Dietary Fiber: 4 g
- Protein: 22 g

Substitutions:

1. If you don't have salmon on hand, you can use any type of protein that you prefer, such as chicken, tofu, or shrimp. Just keep in mind that using a different type of protein may affect the nutritional information.
2. If you don't have sweet potatoes on hand, you can use any type of potato that you prefer, such as russet

potatoes, red potatoes, or yellow potatoes.

3. If you don't have broccoli on hand, you can use any type of vegetables that you prefer, such as asparagus, bell peppers, or zucchini.

GRILLED SHRIMP WITH CORN AND BLACK BEAN SALAD

Servings: 4

Ingredients:

- 1 pound large shrimp, peeled and deveined
- 2 ears of corn, husks removed
- 1 (15-ounce) can black beans, rinsed and drained
- 1 medium tomato, diced
- 1/2 medium red onion, diced
- 1/2 cup chopped fresh cilantro
- 2 tablespoons olive oil
- 2 tablespoons lime juice
- Salt and pepper, to taste

Instructions:

1. Preheat your grill to medium-high heat.
2. Thread the shrimp onto skewers.

3. Grill the shrimp for 2-3 minutes per side, or until they are pink and cooked through.
4. Meanwhile, grill the corn for 10-15 minutes, or until it is tender and slightly charred. Once the corn is cool enough to handle, cut the kernels off the cob.
5. In a large bowl, combine the grilled corn, black beans, tomato, red onion, and cilantro.
6. In a small bowl, whisk together the olive oil, lime juice, salt, and pepper.
7. Pour the dressing over the corn and black bean mixture and toss to combine.
8. Serve the grilled shrimp with the corn and black bean salad on the side.

Health Benefits:

This dish is a good source of protein thanks to the shrimp and black beans. Protein is important for maintaining muscle mass and can help keep you feeling full and satisfied.

The corn and black beans provide a variety of essential vitamins and minerals, as well as fiber, which is important for maintaining good digestive health.

The tomato and red onion add some additional nutrients and flavor to the dish.

Nutritional Information (per serving):

- Calories: 220
- Total Fat: 7 g
- Saturated Fat: 1 g
- Cholesterol: 145 mg
- Sodium: 440 mg
- Total Carbohydrates: 25 g
- Dietary Fiber: 7 g
- Protein: 18 g

Substitutions:

1. If you don't have shrimp on hand, you can use any type of protein that you prefer, such as chicken, tofu, or beef. Just keep in mind that using a different type of protein may affect the nutritional information.
2. If you don't have fresh corn on hand, you can use frozen corn that has been thawed, or canned corn that has been drained and rinsed.
3. If you don't have black beans on hand, you can use any type of beans that you prefer, such as kidney beans, pinto beans, or chickpeas.
4. If you don't have cilantro on hand, you can use any type of fresh herbs that you prefer, such as parsley, basil, or mint. You can also omit the herbs altogether if you prefer.

VEGETABLE AND BEAN SOUP WITH WHOLE GRAIN BREAD

Servings: 4

Ingredients:

- 1 tablespoon olive oil
- 1 medium onion, diced
- 2 cloves garlic, minced
- 2 stalks celery, diced
- 2 carrots, diced
- 1 small zucchini, diced
- 1 (14.5-ounce) can diced tomatoes, undrained
- 1 (15-ounce) can kidney beans, rinsed and drained
- 4 cups low-sodium vegetable broth
- 1 teaspoon Italian seasoning
- Salt and pepper, to taste
- 4 slices whole grain bread

Instructions:

1. Heat the olive oil in a large pot over medium heat.
2. Add the onion and garlic and cook for 3-4 minutes, or until the onion is translucent.
3. Add the celery, carrots, and zucchini to the pot and cook for an additional 5-7 minutes, or until the vegetables are tender.
4. Add the diced tomatoes, kidney beans, vegetable broth, Italian seasoning, salt, and pepper to the pot. Bring the mixture to a boil.
5. Reduce the heat to low and simmer the soup for 15-20 minutes, or until the vegetables are tender.
6. Toast the slices of bread until they are lightly crispy.
7. Serve the soup with the toast on the side.

Health Benefits:

This soup is a good source of fiber thanks to the vegetables and kidney beans. Fiber is important for maintaining good digestive health and can help keep you feeling full and satisfied.
The whole grain bread provides some additional fiber, as well as important vitamins and minerals.
The vegetables in the soup provide a variety of essential vitamins and minerals.

Nutritional Information (per serving):

- Calories: 270
- Total Fat: 5 g
- Saturated Fat: 0.5 g
- Cholesterol: 0 mg
- Sodium: 600 mg
- Total Carbohydrates: 46 g
- Dietary Fiber: 9 g
- Protein: 12 g

Substitutions:

1. If you don't have kidney beans on hand, you can use any type of beans that you prefer, such as black beans, pinto beans, or chickpeas.

2. If you don't have whole grain bread on hand, you can use any type of bread that you prefer, such as white bread, rye bread, or sourdough bread. Just keep in mind that using a bread that is not made with whole grains will not provide the same health benefits.

3. If you don't have zucchini on hand, you can use any type of vegetables that you prefer, such as bell peppers, carrots, or spinach. You can also add additional vegetables to the soup if you prefer.

BAKED CHICKEN WITH QUINOA AND ROASTED VEGETABLES

Servings: 4

Ingredients:

- 4 (4-ounce) chicken breasts
- 1 cup uncooked quinoa
- 2 cups water
- 1 medium zucchini, sliced
- 1 medium bell pepper, sliced
- 1 medium onion, sliced
- 1 tablespoon olive oil
- Salt and pepper, to taste

Instructions:

1. Preheat your oven to 400°F (200°C).
2. Rinse the quinoa in a fine mesh strainer.
3. In a medium saucepan, bring the water to a boil. Add the quinoa and reduce the heat to low.

4. Cover the saucepan and simmer for 15-20 minutes, or until the quinoa is tender and the water is absorbed.
5. Fluff the quinoa with a fork and set it aside.
6. Place the chicken breasts in a baking dish and set aside.
7. In a large bowl, combine the zucchini, bell pepper, and onion. Add the olive oil and season with salt and pepper, to taste.
8. Arrange the vegetables around the chicken in the baking dish.
9. Bake the chicken and vegetables in the preheated oven for 25-30 minutes, or until the chicken is cooked through and the vegetables are tender.
10. Serve the baked chicken with the quinoa and roasted vegetables on the side.

Health Benefits:

This dish is a good source of protein thanks to the chicken and quinoa. Protein is important for maintaining muscle mass and can help keep you feeling full and satisfied.
The vegetables provide a variety of essential vitamins and minerals, as well as fiber, which is important for maintaining good digestive health.
Quinoa is a good source of whole grains, which are important for maintaining good digestive health and can help support a healthy heart.

Nutritional Information (per serving):

- Calories: 310
- Total Fat: 7 g
- Saturated Fat: 1 g
- Cholesterol: 65 mg
- Sodium: 90 mg
- Total Carbohydrates: 36 g

- Dietary Fiber: 5 g
- Protein: 28 g

Substitutions:

1. If you don't have chicken on hand, you can use any type of protein that you prefer, such as tofu, shrimp, or beef. Just keep in mind that using a different type of protein may affect the nutritional information.
2. If you don't have quinoa on hand, you can use any type of grain that you prefer, such as brown rice, wild rice, or farro. Just keep in mind that using a different type of grain may affect the nutritional information.
3. If you don't have zucchini, bell pepper, or onion on hand, you can use any type of vegetables that you prefer. Some options could include mushrooms, asparagus, or eggplant.

GRILLED TURKEY AND VEGETABLE WRAP WITH WHOLE GRAIN TORTILLA

Servings: 4

Ingredients:

- 8 ounces sliced turkey breast
- 4 whole grain tortillas
- 1 cup grated carrot
- 1 cup grated zucchini
- 1 cup grated bell pepper
- 1 cup grated cucumber
- 1/2 cup hummus
- Salt and pepper, to taste

Instructions:

1. Preheat your grill to medium-high heat.

2. Grill the turkey for 2-3 minutes per side, or until it is cooked through and slightly crispy on the outside.
3. In a small bowl, combine the grated carrot, grated zucchini, grated bell pepper, and grated cucumber. Season with salt and pepper, to taste.
4. Spread some hummus on each tortilla.
5. Place some of the grilled turkey and vegetable mixture on one side of each tortilla.
6. Roll up the tortillas and secure them with toothpicks if needed.
7. Grill the wrapped tortillas for 1-2 minutes per side, or until they are crispy and slightly charred.
8. Serve the grilled turkey and vegetable wraps hot.

Health Benefits:

This wrap is a good source of protein thanks to the turkey and hummus. Protein is important for maintaining muscle mass and can help keep you feeling full and satisfied.

The vegetables in the wrap provide a variety of essential vitamins and minerals, as well as fiber, which is important for maintaining good digestive health.

The whole grain tortillas provide some additional fiber, as well as important vitamins and minerals.

Nutritional Information (per serving):

- Calories: 270
- Total Fat: 7 g
- Saturated Fat: 1 g
- Cholesterol: 35 mg
- Sodium: 580 mg
- Total Carbohydrates: 36 g
- Dietary Fiber: 6 g
- Protein: 20 g

Substitutions:

1. If you don't have turkey on hand, you can use any type of protein that you prefer, such as chicken, tofu, or beef. Just keep in mind that using a different type of protein may affect the nutritional information.
2. If you don't have whole grain tortillas on hand, you can use any type of tortillas that you prefer, such as white flour tortillas or corn tortillas. Just keep in mind that using tortillas that are not made with whole grains will not provide the same health benefits.
3. If you don't have hummus on hand, you can use any type of spread that you prefer, such as peanut butter, almond butter, or tahini. You can also omit the spread altogether if you prefer.
4. If you don't have the vegetables called for in the recipe on hand, you can use any type of vegetables that you prefer.

Some options could include sliced mushrooms, grated beetroot, or grated sweet potato.

WHOLE GRAIN PASTA WITH TOMATO SAUCE AND STEAMED VEGETABLES

Servings: 4

Ingredients:

- 8 ounces whole grain pasta
- 1 (24-ounce) jar tomato sauce
- 1 cup steamed broccoli florets
- 1 cup steamed carrot slices
- 1 cup steamed zucchini slices
- Salt and pepper, to taste

Instructions:

1. Bring a large pot of salted water to a boil. Add the pasta and cook according to the package instructions.
2. Meanwhile, heat the tomato sauce in a small saucepan over medium heat.

3. Steam the broccoli, carrot, and zucchini until they are tender.
4. Drain the pasta and return it to the pot.
5. Add the tomato sauce, steamed vegetables, salt, and pepper to the pot with the pasta. Toss to combine.
6. Serve the pasta and vegetables hot.

Health Benefits:

This dish is a good source of fiber thanks to the whole grain pasta and vegetables. Fiber is important for maintaining good digestive health and can help keep you feeling full and satisfied.

The vegetables provide a variety of essential vitamins and minerals.

Whole grain pasta is a good source of complex carbohydrates, which can help provide sustained energy.

Nutritional Information (per serving):

- Calories: 240
- Total Fat: 2 g
- Saturated Fat: 0 g
- Cholesterol: 0 mg
- Sodium: 820 mg
- Total Carbohydrates: 46 g
- Dietary Fiber: 7 g
- Protein: 10 g

Substitutions:

1. If you don't have whole grain pasta on hand, you can use any type of pasta that you prefer, such as white pasta, gluten-free pasta, or legume-based pasta. Just keep in mind that using a pasta that is not made with whole grains will not provide the same health benefits.
2. If you don't have tomato sauce on hand, you can use any type of sauce

that you prefer, such as alfredo sauce, pesto, or a cream-based sauce. You can also make your own sauce by simmering diced tomatoes with some garlic, olive oil, and herbs.

3. If you don't have broccoli, carrot, or zucchini on hand, you can use any type of vegetables that you prefer. Some options could include bell peppers, asparagus, or eggplant.

SLOW COOKER VEGETABLE AND BEAN CHILI WITH WHOLE GRAIN CORNBREAD

Servings: 6

Ingredients:

- 1 tablespoon olive oil
- 1 medium onion, diced
- 2 cloves garlic, minced
- 1 medium bell pepper, diced
- 1 medium zucchini, diced
- 1 (14.5-ounce) can diced tomatoes, undrained
- 1 (15-ounce) can kidney beans, rinsed and drained
- 1 (15-ounce) can black beans, rinsed and drained
- 1 (4-ounce) can diced green chilies, undrained
- 1 cup low-sodium vegetable broth
- 2 tablespoons chili powder

- 1 teaspoon cumin
- 1 teaspoon paprika
- Salt and pepper, to taste
- 1 cup cornmeal
- 1 cup all-purpose flour
- 1 tablespoon baking powder
- 1 cup unsweetened almond milk
- 2 tablespoons honey

Instructions:

1. Heat the olive oil in a large pan over medium heat.
2. Add the onion and garlic and cook for 3-4 minutes, or until the onion is translucent.
3. Add the bell pepper and zucchini to the pan and cook for an additional 5-7 minutes, or until the vegetables are tender.
4. Transfer the vegetables to a slow cooker.
5. Add the diced tomatoes, kidney beans, black beans, green chilies, vegetable

broth, chili powder, cumin, paprika, salt, and pepper to the slow cooker. Stir to combine.

6. Cover the slow cooker and cook on low for 6-8 hours, or until the vegetables are tender and the flavors have melded together.

7. Preheat your oven to 425°F (220°C).

8. In a large bowl, whisk together the cornmeal, flour, and baking powder.

9. Add the almond milk and honey to the dry ingredients and stir until a smooth batter forms.

10. Pour the batter into a greased 9x9-inch baking dish.

11. Bake the cornbread in the preheated oven for 20-25 minutes, or until it is golden brown and a toothpick inserted in the center comes out clean.

12. Serve the vegetable and bean chili with the cornbread on the side.

Health Benefits:

This dish is a good source of protein and fiber thanks to the beans and vegetables. Protein is important for maintaining muscle mass and can help keep you feeling full and satisfied, while fiber is important for maintaining good digestive health.
The vegetables in the chili provide a variety of essential vitamins and minerals.
The cornbread is a good source of whole grains, which are important for maintaining good digestive health and can help support a healthy heart.

Nutritional Information (per serving):

- Calories: 360
- Total Fat: 6 g
- Saturated Fat: 1 g
- Cholesterol: 0 mg
- Sodium: 550 mg
- Total Carbohydrates: 64 g

- Dietary Fiber: 11 g
- Protein: 16 g

Substitutions:

1. If you don't have kidney beans or black beans on hand, you can use any type of beans that you prefer, such as pinto beans

2. If you don't have green chilies on hand, you can omit them or use any type of diced chilies that you prefer. You can also use fresh chilies if you have them on hand.

3. If you don't have almond milk on hand, you can use any type of milk that you prefer, such as cow's milk, soy milk, or oat milk. You can also use water if you prefer.

4. If you don't have honey on hand, you can use any type of sweetener that you prefer, such as agave nectar, maple syrup, or white sugar. You can also

omit the sweetener altogether if you
prefer.

GRILLED PORK CHOP WITH ROASTED POTATOES AND ASPARAGUS

Servings: 4

Ingredients:

- 4 (4-ounce) pork chops
- 4 medium potatoes, cut into 1-inch cubes
- 1 pound asparagus, trimmed
- 1 tablespoon olive oil
- Salt and pepper, to taste

Instructions:

1. Preheat your grill to medium-high heat.
2. Toss the potatoes in some olive oil and season with salt and pepper, to taste.
3. Grill the pork chops for 2-3 minutes per side, or until they are cooked

through and slightly crispy on the outside.

4. Place the potatoes on a sheet pan and roast them in the oven at 400°F (200°C) for 20-25 minutes, or until they are tender and golden brown.
5. Steam the asparagus until it is tender.
6. Serve the grilled pork chop with the roasted potatoes and steamed asparagus on the side.

Health Benefits:

This dish is a good source of protein thanks to the pork chop. Protein is important for maintaining muscle mass and can help keep you feeling full and satisfied.

The potatoes provide some complex carbohydrates, which can help provide sustained energy. They are also a good source of potassium, which is important for maintaining good cardiovascular health.

Asparagus is a good source of fiber, which is important for maintaining good digestive health, as well as a variety of essential vitamins and minerals.

Nutritional Information (per serving):

- Calories: 280
- Total Fat: 9 g
- Saturated Fat: 2.5 g
- Cholesterol: 75 mg
- Sodium: 90 mg
- Total Carbohydrates: 30 g
- Dietary Fiber: 5 g
- Protein: 25 g

Substitutions:

1. If you don't have pork chops on hand, you can use any type of protein that you prefer, such as chicken, beef, or tofu. Just keep in mind that using a different type of protein may affect the nutritional information.

2. If you don't have potatoes on hand, you can use any type of vegetables that you prefer, such as sweet potatoes, carrots, or parsnips. Just keep in mind that using a different type of vegetable may affect the nutritional information.
3. If you don't have asparagus on hand, you can use any type of vegetables that you prefer, such as broccoli, green beans, or bell peppers.

BAKED TOFU WITH BROWN RICE AND STIR-FRIED VEGETABLES

Servings: 4

Ingredients:

- 1 (14-ounce) block tofu
- 2 tablespoons soy sauce
- 1 tablespoon sesame oil
- 2 cups uncooked brown rice
- 4 cups water
- 1 tablespoon olive oil
- 1 medium onion, sliced
- 1 medium bell pepper, sliced
- 1 medium zucchini, sliced
- 1 cup sliced mushrooms
- Salt and pepper, to taste

Instructions:

1. Preheat your oven to 400°F (200°C).
2. Cut the tofu into 1-inch cubes.

3. In a small bowl, whisk together the soy sauce and sesame oil.
4. Place the tofu in a baking dish and pour the soy sauce mixture over the top.
5. Bake the tofu in the preheated oven for 25-30 minutes, or until it is crispy and golden brown.
6. Meanwhile, rinse the brown rice in a fine mesh strainer.
7. In a medium saucepan, bring the water to a boil. Add the brown rice and reduce the heat to low.
8. Cover the saucepan and simmer for 45-50 minutes, or until the rice is tender and the water is absorbed.
9. Fluff the rice with a fork and set it aside.
10. Heat the olive oil in a large pan over medium heat.
11. Add the onion and bell pepper and cook for 3-4 minutes, or until the onion is translucent.

12. Add the zucchini and mushrooms to the pan and cook for an additional 5-7 minutes, or until the vegetables are tender.
13. Season the stir-fried vegetables with salt and pepper, to taste.
14. Serve the baked tofu with the brown rice and stir-fried vegetables on the side.

Health Benefits:

This dish is a good source of protein thanks to the tofu. Protein is important for maintaining muscle mass and can help keep you feeling full and satisfied.

The vegetables provide a variety of essential vitamins and minerals, as well as fiber, which is important for maintaining good digestive health.

Brown rice is a good source of whole grains, which are important for maintaining good digestive health and can help support a healthy heart. It is also a good source of complex carbohydrates, which can help provide sustained energy.

Nutritional Information (per serving):

- Calories: 310
- Fat: 8 g
- Saturated Fat: 1 g
- Cholesterol: 0 mg
- Sodium: 450 mg
- Total Carbohydrates: 45 g
- Dietary Fiber: 4 g
- Protein: 14 g

Substitutions:

1. If you don't have tofu on hand, you can use any type of protein that you prefer, such as chicken, beef, or shrimp. Just keep in mind that using a

different type of protein may affect the nutritional information.

2. If you don't have brown rice on hand, you can use any type of rice that you prefer, such as white rice, wild rice, or quinoa. Just keep in mind that using a different type of rice may affect the nutritional information.

3. If you don't have the vegetables called for in the recipe on hand, you can use any type of vegetables that you prefer. Some options could include broccoli, cauliflower, or peas.

GRILLED CHICKEN CAESAR SALAD WITH WHOLE GRAIN CROUTONS

Servings: 4

Ingredients:

- 4 (4-ounce) chicken breasts
- 1 head romaine lettuce, torn into bite-sized pieces
- 1 cup whole grain croutons
- 1/2 cup grated Parmesan cheese
- 1/2 cup Caesar dressing
- Salt and pepper, to taste

Instructions:

1. Preheat your grill to medium-high heat.
2. Season the chicken breasts with salt and pepper, to taste.
3. Grill the chicken breasts for 6-8 minutes per side, or until they are

cooked through and slightly crispy on the outside.

4. Slice the chicken breasts into thin strips.
5. In a large bowl, toss together the romaine lettuce, croutons, Parmesan cheese, and Caesar dressing.
6. Top the salad with the grilled chicken strips.
7. Serve the salad immediately.

Health Benefits:

This dish is a good source of protein thanks to the chicken and cheese. Protein is important for maintaining muscle mass and can help keep you feeling full and satisfied.
The romaine lettuce provides some fiber, which is important for maintaining good digestive health, as well as a variety of essential vitamins and minerals.
The whole grain croutons provide some complex carbohydrates, which can help provide sustained energy. They are also a

good source of whole grains, which are important for maintaining good digestive health and can help support a healthy heart.

Nutritional Information (per serving):

- Calories: 270
- Total Fat: 15 g
- Saturated Fat: 4 g
- Cholesterol: 75 mg
- Sodium: 400 mg
- Total Carbohydrates: 15 g
- Dietary Fiber: 3 g
- Protein: 25 g

Substitutions:

1. If you don't have chicken breasts on hand, you can use any type of protein that you prefer, such as tofu, shrimp, or beef. Just keep in mind that using a different type of protein may affect the nutritional information.

2. If you don't have romaine lettuce on hand, you can use any type of lettuce that you prefer, such as mixed greens, arugula, or spinach.

3. If you don't have whole grain croutons on hand, you can use any type of croutons that you prefer, such as white bread croutons or gluten-free croutons. You can also omit the croutons altogether if you prefer.

4. If you don't have Caesar dressing on hand, you can use any type of dressing that you prefer, such as ranch dressing, vinaigrette, or Italian dressing. You can also make your own dressing by whisking together some olive oil, lemon juice, Dijon mustard, and garlic.

TURKEY AND VEGETABLE STIR-FRY WITH BROWN RICE

Servings: 4

Ingredients:

- 1 pound ground turkey
- 1 tablespoon olive oil
- 1 medium onion, diced
- 1 medium bell pepper, diced
- 1 medium zucchini, diced
- 1 cup sliced mushrooms
- 2 cloves garlic, minced
- 1 tablespoon soy sauce
- 2 cups uncooked brown rice
- 4 cups water
- Salt and pepper, to taste

Instructions:

1. Heat the olive oil in a large pan over medium heat.

2. Add the ground turkey to the pan and cook for 5-7 minutes, or until it is no longer pink.
3. Add the onion, bell pepper, zucchini, and mushrooms to the pan and cook for an additional 5-7 minutes, or until the vegetables are tender.
4. Stir in the garlic and soy sauce.
5. Rinse the brown rice in a fine mesh strainer.
6. In a medium saucepan, bring the water to a boil. Add the brown rice and reduce the heat to low.
7. Cover the saucepan and simmer for 45-50 minutes, or until the rice is tender and the water is absorbed.
8. Fluff the rice with a fork and set it aside.
9. Serve the turkey and vegetable stir-fry with the brown rice on the side.

Health Benefits:

This dish is a good source of protein thanks to the turkey. Protein is important for maintaining muscle mass and can help keep you feeling full and satisfied.
The vegetables provide a variety of essential vitamins and minerals, as well as fiber, which is important for maintaining good digestive health.
Brown rice is a good source of whole grains, which are important for maintaining good digestive health and can help support a healthy heart. It is also a good source of complex carbohydrates, which can help provide sustained energy.

Nutritional Information (per serving):

- Calories: 360
- Total Fat: 7 g
- Saturated Fat: 1.5 g
- Cholesterol: 75 mg

- Sodium: 420 mg
- Total Carbohydrates: 50 g
- Dietary Fiber: 5 g
- Protein: 25 g

Substitutions:

1. If you don't have ground turkey on hand, you can use any type of protein that you prefer, such as chicken, beef, or tofu. Just keep in mind that using a different type of protein may affect the nutritional information.
2. If you don't have brown rice on hand, you can use any type of rice that you prefer, such as white rice, wild rice, or quinoa. Just keep in mind that using a different type of rice may affect the nutritional information.
3. If you don't have the vegetables called for in the recipe on hand, you can use any type of vegetables that you prefer.

SLOW COOKER BEEF AND VEGETABLE STEW WITH WHOLE GRAIN BISCUITS

Servings: 4

Ingredients:

- 1 pound beef stew meat
- 1 medium onion, diced
- 1 medium carrot, diced
- 1 medium turnip, diced
- 1 medium parsnip, diced
- 1 medium potato, diced
- 2 cloves garlic, minced
- 1 cup beef broth
- 1 cup tomato sauce
- 1 teaspoon paprika
- 1 teaspoon dried thyme
- 1/2 teaspoon salt
- 1/4 teaspoon black pepper
- 1/4 cup all-purpose flour
- 1/4 cup water

- 2 cups whole grain biscuit mix
- 1/2 cup milk

Instructions:

1. Place the beef stew meat, onion, carrot, turnip, parsnip, potato, garlic, beef broth, tomato sauce, paprika, thyme, salt, and black pepper in a slow cooker.
2. Stir the ingredients together until they are well combined.
3. Cover the slow cooker and cook on low heat for 8-10 hours, or until the beef is tender.
4. In a small bowl, whisk together the flour and water.
5. Pour the flour mixture into the slow cooker and stir it into the stew.
6. In a medium bowl, whisk together the biscuit mix and milk.
7. Drop spoonfuls of the biscuit dough on top of the stew.

8. Cover the slow cooker and cook on high heat for an additional 30-40 minutes, or until the biscuits are cooked through and golden brown.
9. Serve the beef and vegetable stew hot, with the biscuits on top.

Health Benefits:

This dish is a good source of protein thanks to the beef. Protein is important for maintaining muscle mass and can help keep you feeling full and satisfied.

The vegetables provide a variety of essential vitamins and minerals, as well as fiber, which is important for maintaining good digestive health.

The whole grain biscuit mix provides some complex carbohydrates, which can help provide sustained energy. It is also a good source of whole grains, which are important for maintaining good digestive health and can help support a healthy heart.

Nutritional Information (per serving):

- Calories: 520
- Total Fat: 16 g
- Saturated Fat: 5 g
- Cholesterol: 75 mg
- Sodium: 920 mg
- Total Carbohydrates: 68 g
- Dietary Fiber: 8 g
- Protein: 32 g

Substitutions:

1. If you don't have beef stew meat on hand, you can use any type of protein that you prefer, such as chicken, pork, or tofu. Just keep in mind that using a different type of protein may affect the nutritional information.
2. If you don't have the vegetables called for in the recipe on hand, you can use any type of vegetables that you prefer.

Some options could include broccoli, cauliflower, or peas.

3. If you don't have whole grain biscuit mix on hand, you can use any type of biscuit mix that you prefer, such as white biscuit mix or gluten-free biscuit mix. You can also make your own biscuit dough by whisking together some all-purpose flour, baking powder, salt, and milk.roccoli, cauliflower, or peas.

GRILLED SALMON WITH QUINOA AND ROASTED VEGETABLES

Servings: 4

Ingredients:

- 4 (4-ounce) salmon fillets
- 1 tablespoon olive oil
- Salt and pepper, to taste
- 1 cup uncooked quinoa
- 2 cups water
- 1 medium zucchini, sliced
- 1 medium yellow squash, sliced
- 1 medium bell pepper, sliced
- 1 medium red onion, sliced
- 1 tablespoon balsamic vinegar

Instructions:

1. Preheat your grill to medium-high heat.

2. Brush the salmon fillets with olive oil and season them with salt and pepper, to taste.

3. Grill the salmon fillets for 6-8 minutes per side, or until they are cooked through and slightly crispy on the outside.

4. Rinse the quinoa in a fine mesh strainer.

5. In a medium saucepan, bring the water to a boil. Add the quinoa and reduce the heat to low.

6. Cover the saucepan and simmer for 15-20 minutes, or until the quinoa is tender and the water is absorbed.

7. Fluff the quinoa with a fork and set it aside.

8. Preheat your oven to 400°F (200°C).

9. On a large baking sheet, toss together the zucchini, yellow squash, bell pepper, and red onion with the balsamic vinegar.

10. Roast the vegetables in the preheated oven for 20-25 minutes, or

until they are tender and slightly caramelized.
11. Serve the grilled salmon with the quinoa and roasted vegetables on the side.

Health Benefits:

This dish is a good source of protein thanks to the salmon. Protein is important for maintaining muscle mass and can help keep you feeling full and satisfied.

The vegetables provide a variety of essential vitamins and minerals, as well as fiber, which is important for maintaining good digestive health.

Quinoa is a good source of plant-based protein and is also a good source of whole grains, which are important for maintaining good digestive health and can help support a healthy heart. It is also a good source of complex carbohydrates, which can help provide sustained energy.

Nutritional Information (per serving):

- Calories: 360
- Total Fat: 13 g
- Saturated Fat: 2 g
- Cholesterol: 75 mg
- Sodium: 120 mg
- Total Carbohydrates: 35 g
- Dietary Fiber: 5 g
- Protein: 28 g

Substitutions:

1. If you don't have salmon on hand, you can use any type of protein that you prefer, such as chicken, tofu, or shrimp. Just keep in mind that using a different type of protein may affect the nutritional information.
2. If you don't have quinoa on hand, you can use any type of grain that you prefer, such as brown rice, wild rice, or farro. Just keep in mind that using a

different type of grain may affect the nutritional information.

3. If you don't have the vegetables called for in the recipe on hand, you can use any type of vegetables that you prefer. Some options could include broccoli, cauliflower, or peas.

BAKED CHICKEN WITH MASHED SWEET POTATOES AND GREEN BEANS

Servings: 4

Ingredients:

- 4 (4-ounce) chicken breasts
- 1 tablespoon olive oil
- Salt and pepper, to taste
- 2 medium sweet potatoes, peeled and cubed
- 1 cup water
- 1/4 cup milk
- 2 tablespoons butter
- 1/2 teaspoon salt
- 1/4 teaspoon black pepper
- 1 cup green beans, trimmed

Instructions:

1. Preheat your oven to 400°F (200°C).

2. Brush the chicken breasts with olive oil and season them with salt and pepper, to taste.
3. Place the chicken breasts on a baking sheet and bake them in the preheated oven for 20-25 minutes, or until they are cooked through and golden brown.
4. While the chicken is baking, place the sweet potatoes in a medium saucepan and add water to cover.
5. Bring the water to a boil, then reduce the heat to low and simmer for 15-20 minutes, or until the sweet potatoes are tender.
6. Drain the sweet potatoes and return them to the saucepan.
7. Add the milk, butter, salt, and pepper to the saucepan and mash the sweet potatoes until they are smooth and creamy.
8. Bring a pot of water to a boil and add the green beans.
9. Cook the green beans for 3-5 minutes, or until they are tender.

10. Drain the green beans and set them aside.
11. Serve the baked chicken with the mashed sweet potatoes and green beans on the side.

Health Benefits:

This dish is a good source of protein thanks to the chicken. Protein is important for maintaining muscle mass and can help keep you feeling full and satisfied.

The sweet potatoes provide a variety of essential vitamins and minerals, as well as fiber, which is important for maintaining good digestive health. They are also a good source of complex carbohydrates, which can help provide sustained energy.

The green beans provide some fiber, as well as a variety of essential vitamins and minerals.

Nutritional Information (per serving):

- Calories: 280
- Total Fat: 12 g
- Saturated Fat: 4 g
- Cholesterol: 75 mg
- Sodium: 360 mg
- Total Carbohydrates: 24 g
- Dietary Fiber: 4 g
- Protein: 22 g

Substitutions:

1. If you don't have chicken breasts on hand, you can use any type of protein that you prefer, such as tofu, shrimp, or beef. Just keep in mind that using a different type of protein may affect the nutritional information.
2. If you don't have sweet potatoes on hand, you can use any type of potato that you prefer, such as white potatoes, red potatoes, or yams. Just

keep in mind that using a different type of potato may affect the nutritional information.

3. If you don't have green beans on hand, you can use any type of vegetable that you prefer. Some options could include broccoli, cauliflower, or peas.

WHOLE GRAIN PIZZA WITH VEGETABLES AND LOW-FAT CHEESE

Servings: 4

Ingredients:

- 1 cup whole grain pizza dough
- 1 tablespoon olive oil
- 1 cup marinara sauce
- 1 medium zucchini, thinly sliced
- 1 medium bell pepper, thinly sliced
- 1 medium onion, thinly sliced
- 1 cup low-fat shredded mozzarella cheese

Instructions:

1. Preheat your oven to 425°F (220°C).
2. On a lightly floured surface, roll out the pizza dough into a 12-inch circle.

3. Place the pizza dough on a baking sheet.

4. Brush the pizza dough with olive oil and spread the marinara sauce over the top.

5. Top the pizza with the zucchini, bell pepper, and onion slices.

6. Sprinkle the cheese over the top of the vegetables.

7. Bake the pizza in the preheated oven for 15-20 minutes, or until the crust is golden brown and the cheese is melted and bubbly.

8. Slice the pizza into 8 wedges and serve hot.

Health Benefits:

This pizza is made with whole grain pizza dough, which is a good source of complex carbohydrates, which can help provide sustained energy. It is also a good source of whole grains, which are important for maintaining good digestive health and can help support a healthy heart.

The vegetables provide a variety of essential vitamins and minerals, as well as fiber, which is important for maintaining good digestive health.

The low-fat cheese provides some protein and calcium, while also being lower in fat than regular cheese.

Nutritional Information (per serving):

- Calories: 220
- Total Fat: 7 g
- Saturated Fat: 2.5 g
- Cholesterol: 10 mg
- Sodium: 500 mg
- Total Carbohydrates: 30 g
- Dietary Fiber: 4 g
- Protein: 10 g

Substitutions:

1. If you don't have whole grain pizza dough on hand, you can use any type of pizza dough that you prefer, such as white pizza dough or gluten-free pizza dough. Just keep in mind that using a different type of pizza dough may affect the nutritional information.
2. If you don't have the vegetables called for in the recipe on hand, you can use any type of vegetables that you prefer. Some options could include broccoli, cauliflower, or peas.
3. If you don't have low-fat mozzarella cheese on hand, you can use any type of cheese that you prefer. Some options could include cheddar, feta, or gorgonzola. Just keep in mind that using a different type of cheese may affect the nutritional information.

GRILLED CHICKEN AND AVOCADO SALAD WITH MIXED GREENS

Servings: 4

Ingredients:

- 4 (4-ounce) chicken breasts
- 1 tablespoon olive oil
- Salt and pepper, to taste
- 1 large avocado, peeled, pitted, and diced
- 1 cup cherry tomatoes, halved
- 1/2 cup crumbled feta cheese
- 4 cups mixed salad greens
- 1/4 cup balsamic vinaigrette

Instructions:

1. Preheat your grill to medium-high heat.
2. Brush the chicken breasts with olive oil and season them with salt and pepper, to taste.

3. Grill the chicken breasts for 6-8
   minutes per side, or until they are
   cooked through and slightly crispy on
   the outside.
4. Slice the chicken breasts into thin
   strips.
5. In a large bowl, toss together the
   chicken, avocado, cherry tomatoes,
   feta cheese, and mixed salad greens.
6. Drizzle the balsamic vinaigrette over
   the top of the salad and toss to coat.
7. Divide the salad among 4 plates and
   serve.

Health Benefits:

This salad is a good source of protein thanks
to the chicken. Protein is important for
maintaining muscle mass and can help keep
you feeling full and satisfied.
The avocado provides a variety of essential
vitamins and minerals, as well as healthy
fats, which can help support a healthy heart.

The mixed salad greens provide a variety of essential vitamins and minerals, as well as fiber, which is important for maintaining good digestive health.

Nutritional Information (per serving):

- Calories: 250
- Total Fat: 16 g
- Saturated Fat: 4 g
- Cholesterol: 75 mg
- Sodium: 380 mg
- Total Carbohydrates: 12 g
- Dietary Fiber: 6 g
- Protein: 20 g

Substitutions:

1. If you don't have chicken breasts on hand, you can use any type of protein that you prefer, such as tofu, shrimp, or beef. Just keep in mind that using a

different type of protein may affect the nutritional information.

2. If you don't have avocado on hand, you can omit it or use any type of fruit or vegetable that you prefer. Some options could include mango, papaya, or cucumber.

3. If you don't have cherry tomatoes on hand, you can use any type of tomato that you prefer, or omit them altogether.

4. If you don't have feta cheese on hand, you can use any type of cheese that you prefer. Some options could include cheddar, gorgonzola, or goat cheese. Just keep in mind that using a different type of cheese may affect the nutritional information.

5. If you don't have balsamic vinaigrette on any type of salad dressing that you prefer. Some options could include ranch, Caesar, or honey mustard. Just keep in mind that using a different

type of salad dressing may affect the
nutritional information.

SLOW COOKER CHICKEN AND VEGETABLE SOUP WITH WHOLE GRAIN BREAD

Servings: 6

Ingredients:

- 1 pound chicken breasts
- 1 tablespoon olive oil
- Salt and pepper, to taste
- 1 medium onion, chopped
- 2 cloves garlic, minced
- 2 medium carrots, chopped
- 2 stalks celery, chopped
- 1 medium zucchini, chopped
- 1 (14.5-ounce) can diced tomatoes
- 4 cups chicken broth
- 1 cup water
- 1 teaspoon dried oregano
- 1 teaspoon dried basil
- 1/2 teaspoon salt
- 1/4 teaspoon black pepper

- 6 slices whole grain bread

Instructions:

1. Heat a large skillet over medium heat.
2. Add the chicken breasts and cook for 6-8 minutes per side, or until they are cooked through and golden brown.
3. Remove the chicken from the skillet and set it aside to cool.
4. Once the chicken is cool, shred it into bite-sized pieces.
5. In the same skillet, heat the olive oil over medium heat.
6. Add the onion, garlic, carrots, and celery to the skillet and cook for 5-7 minutes, or until they are tender.
7. Transfer the vegetables to a slow cooker.
8. Add the zucchini, diced tomatoes, chicken broth, water, oregano, basil, salt, and pepper to the slow cooker.
9. Stir to combine.

10.   Place the shredded chicken in the slow cooker.
11. Cover the slow cooker and cook on low for 8-10 hours, or on high for 4-6 hours.
12. Serve the soup with a slice of whole grain bread on the side.

Health Benefits:

This soup is a good source of protein thanks to the chicken. Protein is important for maintaining muscle mass and can help keep you feeling full and satisfied.

The vegetables provide a variety of essential vitamins and minerals, as well as fiber, which is important for maintaining good digestive health.

The whole grain bread provides some protein and fiber, as well as complex carbohydrates, which can help provide sustained energy. It is also a good source of whole grains, which are important for maintaining good digestive health and can help support a healthy heart.

Nutritional Information (per serving):

- Calories: 260
- Total Fat: 7 g
- Saturated Fat: 1.5 g
- Cholesterol: 55 mg
- Sodium: 640 mg
- Total Carbohydrates: 32 g
- Dietary Fiber: 5 g
- Protein: 20 g

Substitutions:

1. If you don't have chicken breasts on hand, you can use any type of protein that you prefer, such as tofu, shrimp, or beef. Just keep in mind that using a different type of protein may affect the nutritional information.

2. If you don't have any of the vegetables
   called for in the recipe on hand, you
   can use any type of vegetables that you
   prefer. Some options could include
   broccoli, cauliflower, or peas.

3. If you don't have whole grain bread on
   hand, you can use any type of bread
   that you prefer, such as white bread,
   rye bread, or gluten-free bread. Just
   keep in mind that using a different
   type of bread may affect the
   nutritional information.

BAKED TILAPIA WITH QUINOA AND STEAMED BROCCOLI

Servings: 4

Ingredients:

1. 4 (4-ounce) tilapia fillets
2. 1 tablespoon olive oil
3. Salt and pepper, to taste
4. 1 cup uncooked quinoa
5. 2 cups water
6. 1/2 teaspoon salt
7. 1/4 teaspoon black pepper
8. 1 pound broccoli florets

Instructions:

1. Preheat your oven to 400°F (200°C).
2. Brush the tilapia fillets with olive oil and season them with salt and pepper, to taste.
3. Place the tilapia fillets on a baking sheet and bake them in the preheated

oven for 12-15 minutes, or until they are cooked through and flaky.

4. While the tilapia is baking, rinse the quinoa in a fine-mesh sieve.
5. In a medium saucepan, bring the water to a boil.
6. Add the quinoa, salt, and pepper to the saucepan.
7. Reduce the heat to low and simmer the quinoa for 15-20 minutes, or until the water has been absorbed and the quinoa is tender.
8. Bring a pot of water to a boil and add the broccoli florets.
9. Cook the broccoli for 3-5 minutes, or until it is tender.
10. Drain the broccoli and set it aside.
11. Serve the baked tilapia with the quinoa and steamed broccoli on the side.

Health Benefits:

This dish is a good source of protein thanks to the tilapia. Protein is important for maintaining muscle mass and can help keep you feeling full and satisfied.

The quinoa provides a variety of essential vitamins and minerals, as well as fiber, which is important for maintaining good digestive health. It is also a good source of complex carbohydrates, which can help provide sustained energy.

The broccoli provides a variety of essential vitamins and minerals, as well as fiber, which is important for maintaining good digestive health. It is also a good source of antioxidants, which can help support a healthy immune system.

Nutritional Information (per serving):

1. Calories: 300
2. Total Fat: 8 g

3. Saturated Fat: 1 g
4. Cholesterol: 45 mg
5. Sodium: 260 mg
6. Total Carbohydrates: 35 g
7. Dietary Fiber: 5 g
8. Protein: 25 g

Substitutions:

1. If you don't have tilapia on hand, you can use any type of fish that you prefer, such as salmon or cod. Just keep in mind that using a different type of fish may affect the nutritional information.

2. If you don't have quinoa on hand, you can use any type of grain that you prefer, such as rice, pasta, or oats. Just keep in mind that using a different type of grain may affect the nutritional information.

3. If you don't have broccoli on hand, you can use any type of vegetable that you prefer. Some options could

include peas, asparagus, or green
beans.

GRILLED PORK WITH ROASTED SWEET POTATO AND BRUSSELS SPROUTS

Servings: 4

Ingredients:

- 1 pound pork tenderloin
- 1 tablespoon olive oil
- Salt and pepper, to taste
- 2 medium sweet potatoes, peeled and cut into 1-inch cubes
- 1 pound Brussels sprouts, trimmed and halved
- 1 tablespoon balsamic vinegar

Instructions:

1. Preheat your grill to medium-high heat.

2. Brush the pork tenderloin with olive oil and season it with salt and pepper, to taste.
3. Grill the pork tenderloin for 6-8 minutes per side, or until it is cooked through and slightly crispy on the outside.
4. Slice the pork tenderloin into thin slices.
5. Preheat your oven to 400°F (200°C).
6. On a large baking sheet, toss the sweet potato cubes and Brussels sprouts with the balsamic vinegar.
7. Roast the sweet potatoes and Brussels sprouts in the preheated oven for 20-25 minutes, or until they are tender and slightly caramelized.
8. Serve the grilled pork with the roasted sweet potatoes and Brussels sprouts on the side.

Health Benefits:

This dish is a good source of protein thanks to the pork. Protein is important for maintaining muscle mass and can help keep you feeling full and satisfied.

The sweet potatoes provide a variety of essential vitamins and minerals, as well as fiber, which is important for maintaining good digestive health. They are also a good source of complex carbohydrates, which can help provide sustained energy.

The Brussels sprouts provide a variety of essential vitamins and minerals, as well as fiber, which is important for maintaining good digestive health. They are also a good source of antioxidants, which can help support a healthy immune system.

Nutritional Information (per serving):

- Calories: 260
- Total Fat: 8 g
- Saturated Fat: 2.5 g
- Cholesterol: 75 mg

- Sodium: 120 mg
- Total Carbohydrates: 25 g
- Dietary Fiber: 4 g
- Protein: 25 g

Substitutions:

1. If you don't have pork tenderloin on hand, you can use any type of pork that you prefer, such as pork chops or pork loin. Just keep in mind that using a different type of pork may affect the nutritional information.
2. If you don't have sweet potatoes on hand, you can use any type of potato that you prefer, such as regular potatoes, yams, or sweet potatoes.
3. If you don't have Brussels sprouts on hand, you can use any type of vegetable that you prefer. Some options could include broccoli, cauliflower, or peas.

VEGETABLE AND BEAN BURRITOS WITH WHOLE GRAIN TORTILLAS

Servings: 4

Ingredients:

- 4 whole grain tortillas
- 1 cup cooked black beans
- 1 cup cooked brown rice
- 1 cup diced bell peppers
- 1 cup diced onions
- 1 cup diced tomatoes
- 1 cup shredded lettuce
- 1 cup shredded cheese (optional)
- Salsa, to taste (optional)

Instructions:

1. Heat a large skillet over medium heat.
2. Add the black beans, brown rice, bell peppers, onions, and tomatoes to the skillet.

3. Cook the vegetables and beans for 5-7 minutes, or until they are tender.
4. Warm the tortillas in a separate skillet over medium heat for 30 seconds on each side.
5. Divide the vegetable and bean mixture among the tortillas.
6. Top the tortillas with the shredded lettuce and shredded cheese, if using.
7. Roll the tortillas up tightly and slice them in half.
8. Serve the burritos with salsa on the side, if desired.

Health Benefits:

This dish is a good source of protein thanks to the black beans. Protein is important for maintaining muscle mass and can help keep you feeling full and satisfied.

The whole grain tortillas provide some protein and fiber, as well as complex carbohydrates, which can help provide sustained energy. They are also a good source of whole grains, which are important for maintaining good digestive health and can help support a healthy heart.

The vegetables provide a variety of essential vitamins and minerals, as well as fiber, which is important for maintaining good digestive health.

Nutritional Information (per serving):

- Calories: 300
- Total Fat: 5 g
- Saturated Fat: 2 g
- Cholesterol: 15 mg
- Sodium: 270 mg
- Total Carbohydrates: 53 g
- Dietary Fiber: 10 g
- Protein: 13 g

Substitutions:

1. If you don't have black beans on hand, you can use any type of bean that you

prefer, such as kidney beans, pinto beans, or chickpeas. Just keep in mind that using a different type of bean may affect the nutritional information.

2. If you don't have brown rice on hand, you can use any type of grain that you prefer, such as quinoa, oats, or pasta. Just keep in mind that using a different type of grain may affect the nutritional information.

3. If you don't have bell peppers on hand, you can use any type of vegetable that you prefer. Some options could include onions, mushrooms, or zucchini.

4. If you don't have whole grain tortillas on hand, you can use any type of tortilla that you prefer, such as white flour tortillas or corn tortillas. Just keep in mind that using a different type of tortilla may affect the nutritional information.

GRILLED CHICKEN AND VEGETABLE SKEWERS WITH BROWN RICE

Servings: 4

Ingredients:

- 1 pound chicken breasts, cut into 1-inch cubes
- 1 tablespoon olive oil
- Salt and pepper, to taste
- 1 medium bell pepper, cut into 1-inch pieces
- 1 medium onion, cut into 1-inch pieces
- 1 medium zucchini, cut into 1-inch slices
- 1 cup uncooked brown rice
- 2 cups water
- 1/2 teaspoon salt

Instructions:

1. Preheat your grill to medium-high heat.
2. Thread the chicken cubes, bell pepper, onion, and zucchini onto skewers.
3. Brush the skewers with olive oil and season them with salt and pepper, to taste.
4. Grill the skewers for 6-8 minutes per side, or until the chicken is cooked through and the vegetables are tender.
5. While the skewers are grilling, rinse the brown rice in a fine-mesh sieve.
6. In a medium saucepan, bring the water to a boil.
7. Add the brown rice, salt, and pepper to the saucepan.
8. Reduce the heat to low and simmer the rice for 35-45 minutes, or until the water has been absorbed and the rice is tender.

9. Serve the grilled chicken and vegetable skewers with the brown rice on the side.

Health Benefits:

This dish is a good source of protein thanks to the chicken. Protein is important for maintaining muscle mass and can help keep you feeling full and satisfied.

The brown rice provides a variety of essential vitamins and minerals, as well as fiber, which is important for maintaining good digestive health. It is also a good source of complex carbohydrates, which can help provide sustained energy.

The vegetables provide a variety of essential vitamins and minerals, as well as fiber, which is important for maintaining good digestive health.

Nutritional Information (per serving):

- Calories: 280
- Total Fat: 6 g
- Saturated Fat: 1 g
- Cholesterol: 75 mg
- Sodium: 270 mg
- Total Carbohydrates: 36 g
- Dietary Fiber: 4 g
- Protein: 25 g

Substitutions:

1. If you don't have chicken breasts on hand, you can use any type of protein that you prefer, such as tofu, shrimp, or beef. Just keep in mind that using a different type of protein may affect the nutritional information.
2. If you don't have bell peppers on hand, you can use any type of vegetable that you prefer. Some

options could include onions, mushrooms, or zucchini.

3. If you don't have brown rice on hand, you can use any type of grain that you prefer, such as quinoa, oats, or pasta. Just keep in mind that using a different type of grain may affect the nutritional information.

BAKED TURKEY MEATLOAF WITH MASHED SWEET POTATOES AND GREEN BEANS

Servings: 4

Ingredients:

- 1 pound ground turkey
- 1/2 cup breadcrumbs
- 1 egg, beaten
- 1/4 cup diced onions
- 1/4 cup diced bell peppers
- 1 tablespoon Worcestershire sauce
- Salt and pepper, to taste
- 2 medium sweet potatoes, peeled and cut into 1-inch cubes
- 1 pound green beans, trimmed
- 2 tablespoons butter
- 1/4 cup milk

Instructions:

1. Preheat your oven to 350°F (180°C).
2. In a large mixing bowl, combine the ground turkey, breadcrumbs, egg, onions, bell peppers, Worcestershire sauce, salt, and pepper.
3. Shape the mixture into a loaf and place it in a baking dish.
4. Bake the turkey meatloaf in the preheated oven for 45-55 minutes, or until it is cooked through and the internal temperature reaches 165°F (74°C).
5. While the meatloaf is baking, bring a pot of water to a boil and add the sweet potato cubes.
6. Cook the sweet potatoes for 10-15 minutes, or until they are tender.
7. Drain the sweet potatoes and add them to a large mixing bowl.
8. Add the butter and milk to the sweet potatoes and mash them until they are smooth and creamy.

9. Bring another pot of water to a boil and add the green beans.
10. Cook the green beans for 3-5 minutes, or until they are tender.
11. Drain the green beans and set them aside.
12. Serve the baked turkey meatloaf with the mashed sweet potatoes and green beans on the side.

Health Benefits:

This dish is a good source of protein thanks to the ground turkey. Protein is important for maintaining muscle mass and can help keep you feeling full and satisfied.

The sweet potatoes provide a variety of essential vitamins and minerals, as well as fiber, which is important for maintaining good digestive health. They are also a good source of complex carbohydrates, which can help provide sustained energy.

The green beans provide a variety of essential vitamins and minerals, as well as fiber, which is important for maintaining good digestive health. They are also a good source of antioxidants, which can help support a healthy immune system.

Nutritional Information (per serving):

- Calories: 320
- Total Fat: 12 g
- Saturated Fat: 4 g
- Cholesterol: 110 mg
- Sodium: 410 mg
- Total Carbohydrates: 32 g
- Dietary Fiber: 4 g
- Protein: 25 g

Substitutions:

1. If you don't have ground turkey on hand, you can use any type of protein that you prefer, such as beef, chicken, or pork. Just keep in mind that using a

different type of protein may affect the nutritional information.

2. If you don't have breadcrumbs on hand, you can use any type of binder that you prefer, such as oats, cracker crumbs, or crushed cereal.

3. If you don't have bell peppers on hand, you can use any type of vegetable that you prefer. Some options could include onions, mushrooms, or zucchini.

4. If you don't have sweet potatoes on hand, you can use any type of potato that you prefer, such as regular potatoes, yams, or sweet potatoes.

5. If you don't have green beans on hand, you can use any type of vegetable that you prefer. Some options could include broccoli, cauliflower, or peas.

GRILLED SALMON WITH QUINOA AND ROASTED ASPARAGUS

Servings: 4

Ingredients:

- 1 pound salmon fillets
- 1 tablespoon olive oil
- Salt and pepper, to taste
- 1 cup uncooked quinoa
- 2 cups water
- 1/2 teaspoon salt
- 1 pound asparagus, trimmed

Instructions:

1. Preheat your grill to medium-high heat.
2. Brush the salmon fillets with olive oil and season them with salt and pepper, to taste.
3. Grill the salmon fillets for 6-8 minutes per side, or until they are cooked

through and slightly crispy on the outside.

4. While the salmon is grilling, rinse the quinoa in a fine-mesh sieve.
5. In a medium saucepan, bring the water to a boil.
6. Add the quinoa, salt, and pepper to the saucepan.
7. Reduce the heat to low and simmer the quinoa for 20-25 minutes, or until the water has been absorbed and the quinoa is tender.
8. Preheat your oven to 400°F (200°C).
9. On a large baking sheet, toss the asparagus with olive oil and season it with salt and pepper, to taste.
10. Roast the asparagus in the preheated oven for 10-15 minutes, or until it is tender and slightly caramelized.
11. Serve the grilled salmon with the quinoa and roasted asparagus on the side.

Health Benefits:

This dish is a good source of protein thanks to the salmon. Protein is important for maintaining muscle mass and can help keep you feeling full and satisfied. Salmon is also a good source of omega-3 fatty acids, which can help support a healthy heart.
The quinoa provides a variety of essential vitamins and minerals, as well as fiber, which is important for maintaining good digestive health. It is also a good source of protein and complex carbohydrates, which can help provide sustained energy.
The asparagus provides a variety of essential vitamins and minerals, as well as fiber, which is important for maintaining good digestive health. Asparagus is also a good source of antioxidants, which can help support a healthy immune system.

Nutritional Information (per serving):

- Calories: 360
- Total Fat: 12 g
- Saturated Fat: 2 g
- Cholesterol: 75 mg
- Sodium: 260 mg
- Total Carbohydrates: 36 g
- Dietary Fiber: 5 g
- Protein: 26 g

Substitutions:

1. If you don't have salmon on hand, you can use any type of protein that you prefer, such as chicken, beef, or pork. Just keep in mind that using a different type of protein may affect the nutritional information.
2. If you don't have quinoa on hand, you can use any type of grain that you prefer, such as brown rice, oats, or pasta. Just keep in mind that using a

different type of grain may affect the nutritional information.

3. If you don't have asparagus on hand, you can use any type of vegetable that you prefer. Some options could include broccoli, cauliflower, or peas.

CONCLUSION

As you turn the final page of this cookbook, we hope that the journey through its pages has been a fulfilling and enlightening one. Living with diabetes and kidney disease can be a challenging and at times, overwhelming experience. But with the right tools and resources, it is possible to manage your health and enjoy delicious meals that nourish both your body and soul.

We understand the difficulties that come with managing a diabetes and renal diet and that is why we have created this cookbook to offer you a wealth of recipes that are not only delicious and satisfying, but also tailored to meet your specific dietary needs. We hope that you have found new inspiration and ideas for meals that will make it easier to follow your diet while still enjoying the pleasures of food.

We hope that you have found the recipes and tips in this cookbook helpful and that they have made a positive impact in your life. Remember, every meal is an opportunity to take care of yourself and celebrate the gift of good health. Eating should be a source of pleasure and nourishment, not a source of stress or frustration. We encourage you to continue to experiment and discover new flavors and ingredients that will help make your meals even more enjoyable.

We want to thank you for joining us on this journey, for trusting in our expertise and for choosing this cookbook as a guide to help you manage your diabetes and kidney disease. We are honored to be a part of your health journey, and we are here to support you every step of the way. We wish you all the best on your path to wellness and hope that the recipes and tips in this cookbook will continue to serve you well for many years to come.